# METABOLIC DIET PLAN AND EXERCISE FOR ENDOMORPH

Secrets to boost Metabolism, quick weight loss, optimal health with delicious recipes

SARAH BILLY

Copyright © 2024 – **Sarah Billy**

ISBN:

Printed in the United States of America

**Disclaimer**

All rights reserved. No part of this publication may be reproduced, distributed, or transmitted in any form or by any means, including photocopying, recording, or other electronic or mechanical methods, without the prior written permission of the publisher, except in the case of brief quotations embodied in critical reviews and certain other non-commercial uses permitted by copyright law. For permission requests, write to the publisher, addressed at the address below

## Table of Contents

**Table of Contents ............................................. 3**

**Introduction ................................................. 10**

    Understanding the Endomorphic Metabolism ................................................. 10

    The Science Behind Resetting Metabolics for Endomorphs ................................................. 13

**Assessing Your Metabolic Blueprint .......... 16**

    Identifying Endomorphic Traits ..................... 16

    Metabolic Rate Assessment and Setting Realistic Goals ............................................. 19

**The Resetting Nutrition Plan ......................... 23**

    Principles of Endomorphic Nutrition: .......... 23

    The Role of Nutrient Timing in Boosting Metabolism ................................................. 27

    Meal Frequency and Portion Control Strategies ................................................. 31

**Resetting Metabolic Workout Protocols .... 36**

Exercise Routines for Endomorphic Bodies 36

Cardiovascular Exercise: ............................ 36

Strength Training: ....................................... 38

Flexibility and Mobility: .............................. 39

Abdominal Training: .................................. 40

Post-Workout Recovery ............................ 41

Consistency and Progress: ....................... 41

Holistic Approach: ..................................... 42

Professional Guidance: ............................. 42

High-Intensity Interval Training (HIIT) for Metabolic Acceleration ............................. 43

Strength Training Techniques for Sculpting and Toning .................................................. 48

## 4 weeks Meal Plan for Building Your Metabolic ......................................................... 56

Week 1 ....................................................... 56

Week 2 ....................................................... 60

Week 3 ......................................................... 65

Week 4 ......................................................... 70

**Metabolic Breakfast Boosters Recipes ...... 75**

Protein-Packed Omelet ............................... 75

Quinoa Breakfast Bowl ................................ 76

Avocado Toast with Poached Eggs .......... 77

Chia Seed Pudding Parfait ........................ 78

Spinach and Mushroom Breakfast Wrap ... 79

Blueberry Protein Smoothie ........................ 81

Sweet Potato Hash with Turkey Sausage ... 82

Cottage Cheese and Pineapple Bowl ...... 83

Egg and Veggie Breakfast Burrito .............. 84

Peanut Butter Banana Toast ....................... 85

Salmon and Avocado Bagel ...................... 86

Mango Coconut Overnight Oats ............... 87

Turkey and Spinach Breakfast Muffins ....... 88

Raspberry Almond Chia Pudding .............. 89

Green Tea Smoothie .................................... 90

**Metabolic Lunchtime Power Recipes ....... 92**

Grilled Chicken and Quinoa Salad............ 92

Salmon and Avocado Wrap ...................... 93

Mediterranean Chickpea Salad ................ 94

Turkey and Quinoa Stuffed Peppers .......... 95

Whole-grain pasta with Pesto and Veggies
................................................................. 96

Shrimp and Quinoa Bowl ............................ 98

Vegetarian Chickpea Stir-Fry..................... 99

Tuna Salad Stuffed Avocado ................... 100

Eggplant and Lentil Curry ......................... 101

Chicken and Vegetable Quinoa Bowl.... 102

Sweet Potato and Black Bean Quesadilla
............................................................... 103

Caprese Salad with Grilled Chicken........ 104

Lentil and Vegetable Soup....................... 106

Turkey and Quinoa Stuffed Acorn Squash .................................................................. 107

Asian-Inspired Tofu Stir-Fry ......................... 108

**Metabolic Dinner Delights Recipes ......... 109**

Grilled Salmon with Lemon-Dill Sauce ..... 109

Quinoa and Vegetable Stuffed Bell Peppers .................................................................. 110

Chicken and Broccoli Stir-Fry ..................... 111

Vegetarian Lentil Soup ............................... 112

Mushroom and Spinach Stuffed Chicken Breast ........................................................ 113

Sweet Potato and Chickpea Curry .......... 114

Baked Cod with Mediterranean Salsa ..... 115

Vegetable and Tofu Stir-Fry ....................... 116

Spinach and Feta-Stuffed Chicken Thighs .................................................................. 117

Lemon Herb Grilled Shrimp ....................... 119

Veggie-Packed Turkey Chili ...................... 120

Cauliflower and Chickpea Curry ............. 121

Sesame Ginger Beef Stir-Fry ..................... 122

Pesto Zoodles with Grilled Chicken .......... 123

**Metabolic Snack Smart Recipes ............. 124**

Almond Butter Banana Bites ..................... 124

Cucumber and Hummus ........................... 125

Hard-Boiled Eggs with Avocado .............. 125

Trail Mix ..................................................... 126

Apple Slices with Peanut Butter ................ 127

Rice Cake with Cottage Cheese and Pineapple ................................................... 128

Kale Chips ................................................. 129

Cherry Tomatoes with Mozzarella ........... 129

Carrot Sticks with Hummus ....................... 130

Cottage Cheese and Mango Salsa ........ 131

Stuffed Dates with Almond Butter ............ 132

Whole Grain Crackers with Tuna Salad ... 133

Yogurt-Dipped Strawberries ....................... 134

Pumpkin Seeds and Dried Apricots .......... 135

**Conclusion................................................... 136**

# Chapter 1

# Introduction

## Understanding the Endomorphic Metabolism

Endomorphs typically have a body composition characterized by a higher percentage of body fat and a tendency to store excess calories as fat rather than burn them for energy. The metabolism of endomorphs is often regarded as slower compared to other body types, presenting unique challenges in achieving and maintaining a healthy weight.

One defining feature of endomorphic metabolism is a propensity to gain weight easily, especially in the form of fat, even with relatively lower caloric intake. This can be attributed to genetic factors that influence how the body processes and stores energy.

Endomorphs typically have a rounder or softer physique, and they may find it challenging to shed excess weight through traditional diet and exercise alone.

Metabolism in endomorphs is influenced by hormonal factors, including insulin sensitivity and the body's response to certain foods. Endomorphs often exhibit higher insulin levels, which can contribute to the storage of excess calories as fat. Understanding and managing insulin levels become crucial for optimizing the endomorphic metabolism.

The metabolic rate, or the rate at which the body burns calories at rest, is another aspect that distinguishes endomorphs. While it may be slower compared to other body types, it's essential to avoid misconceptions and recognize that individual metabolic rates can vary widely within the endomorphic category. Factors such as age, muscle mass, and overall health play significant roles in influencing metabolic rate.

Despite the challenges, endomorphs have unique strengths. They tend to build muscle relatively easily, and a well-designed fitness and nutrition plan can leverage this quality to boost metabolism and support fat loss. Strategies for endomorphic individuals should focus on a balanced and nutrient-dense diet, incorporating regular physical activity that includes both cardiovascular exercises and strength training. Additionally, managing stress levels and getting adequate sleep are essential components of optimizing the endomorphic metabolism.

In essence, understanding the endomorphic metabolism involves recognizing its nuances and adopting tailored approaches that align with the body's natural tendencies. By embracing personalized strategies, individuals with an endomorphic body type can achieve and maintain their health and fitness goals effectively.

## The Science Behind Resetting Metabolics for Endomorphs

This revolves around optimizing metabolic processes to enhance energy expenditure, promote fat loss, and improve overall body composition. Endomorphs typically face challenges related to a slower metabolism, increased insulin sensitivity, and a predisposition to store excess calories as fat. Metabolic Rejuvenation aims to address these factors through targeted interventions.

One key aspect of the science behind metabolic Rejuvenation is the recognition of the impact of insulin on fat storage. Endomorphs often have higher insulin levels, which can lead to more efficient fat storage.

Metabolic Rejuvenation focuses on balancing blood sugar levels through dietary modifications, emphasizing complex carbohydrates, fiber, and lean proteins to manage insulin responses effectively.

Moreover, incorporating strategic exercise routines is fundamental to the reset for endomorphs. High-intensity interval Training (HIIT) and strength training play pivotal roles in boosting metabolism, promoting calorie burn, and enhancing muscle development. Muscle, being metabolically active, contributes to increased energy expenditure, even at rest.

Nutrient timing and meal frequency are integral components of the reset. Eating smaller, well-balanced meals throughout the day helps maintain stable blood sugar levels and prevents overeating, supporting metabolic efficiency.

Additionally, stress management is a crucial element. Elevated stress levels can contribute to hormonal imbalances that affect metabolism negatively. Techniques such as mindfulness, meditation, and adequate sleep are incorporated into the reset plan to mitigate stress-related impacts.

## Chapter 2

## Assessing Your Metabolic Blueprint

### Identifying Endomorphic Traits

Endomorphs tend to exhibit traits that make them prone to storing excess fat and facing challenges in achieving and maintaining a lean physique.

Here are key endomorphic traits:

1. **Rounder Body Shape:**

    - Endomorphs typically have a softer, rounder physique characterized by a curvier and more voluptuous appearance. Weight is often distributed around the abdomen, hips, and thighs.

2. **Higher Percentage of Body Fat:**

    - Individuals with an endomorphic body type naturally carry a higher percentage of body fat. Fat tends to accumulate easily, especially in areas like the waist and hips.

3. **Slower Metabolism:**

    - Endomorphs may experience a slower metabolic rate compared to other body types. This means they may burn calories at a slightly lower rate, making it challenging to lose weight through conventional diet and exercise alone.

4. **Tendency to Gain Weight Easily:**

    - One of the hallmark traits of endomorphs is a propensity to gain weight easily. Even with a moderate caloric intake, they may find it challenging to prevent weight gain.

5. **Difficulty Losing Weight:**
    - Weight loss can be more challenging for endomorphs. They often need to adopt specific strategies that consider their unique metabolic profile, including a focus on both nutrition and exercise.

6. **Muscle Development:**
    - Endomorphs tend to have a natural predisposition for building muscle. While this can be an advantage, it also means that without proper management, they may develop a bulky appearance.

7. **Insulin Sensitivity:**
    - Endomorphs often display higher insulin sensitivity, contributing to more efficient fat storage. This underscores the importance of managing blood sugar levels through dietary choices.

8. **Preference for Carbohydrates:**
    - Endomorphs may have a preference for carbohydrate-rich foods. While this can provide quick energy, it's crucial to focus on the quality and quantity of carbohydrates to support overall health.

## Metabolic Rate Assessment and Setting Realistic Goals

The metabolic rate, often measured in terms of Basal Metabolic Rate (BMR) and Total Daily

Energy Expenditure (TDEE), provides insights into the number of calories the body requires at rest and during daily activities.

For endomorphs, who may experience a slower metabolic rate, assessing and understanding their baseline metabolism is essential. Techniques like indirect calorimetry measure the oxygen consumption and carbon dioxide production during rest, aiding in the calculation of BMR. This baseline figure reflects the minimum calories needed to maintain bodily functions while at rest. Factoring in daily activities, such as work, exercise, and daily tasks, gives a more comprehensive picture of TDEE, which represents the total calories burned in a day.

Setting realistic goals based on metabolic rate involves a balanced and personalized approach. A modest caloric deficit, where calories consumed are slightly lower than calories expended, is often recommended for weight loss. However, the deficit should be sustainable and not overly restrictive to ensure nutritional needs are met and energy levels are maintained. The focus extends beyond the scale; it includes improving overall body composition, enhancing metabolic health, and building sustainable habits.

Realistic goals for endomorphs involve acknowledging that changes may take time. Aiming for a gradual weight loss of 1-2 pounds per week is realistic and aligns with a healthy and sustainable approach. Incorporating strength training into the fitness routine is beneficial, as it not only aids in fat loss but also promotes muscle development, which contributes to an elevated metabolic rate over time.

Furthermore, setting goals that go beyond weight loss metrics, such as achieving a certain body fat percentage or completing specific fitness milestones, enhances the overall health and wellness journey. Embracing a holistic approach that considers factors like stress management, sleep, and overall well-being ensures a comprehensive strategy for endomorphs to achieve and maintain their health and fitness goals over the long term. By understanding their metabolic rate and setting realistic, multifaceted goals, individuals can embark on a transformative journey that prioritizes both physical and mental well-being.

## Chapter 3

## The Resetting Nutrition Plan

**Principles of Endomorphic Nutrition:**

Principles of endomorphic nutrition revolve around adopting a dietary approach that aligns with the unique characteristics of individuals with an endomorphic body type. Endomorphs often face challenges related to higher body fat storage and a slower metabolic rate, necessitating a tailored nutritional strategy. Here are key principles for endomorphic nutrition:

1. **Balanced Macronutrient Intake:**

Endomorphs benefit from a balanced intake of macronutrients—protein, carbohydrates, and fats. Prioritizing lean protein sources supports muscle development while incorporating complex carbohydrates and healthy fats helps maintain steady energy levels.

2. **Focus on Quality Carbohydrates:**

Choose complex carbohydrates with a low glycemic index to manage blood sugar levels effectively. Whole grains, vegetables, and legumes provide sustained energy and minimize the risk of excessive fat storage associated with insulin spikes.

3. **Moderate Caloric Intake:**

While creating a modest caloric deficit is essential for weight management, overly restrictive diets should be avoided. A moderate reduction in calories supports fat loss without compromising nutritional needs or triggering metabolic adaptations.

4. **Frequent, Smaller Meals:**

Eating smaller, balanced meals throughout the day helps regulate blood sugar levels and prevents overeating. This approach supports a more stable metabolic rate and minimizes the likelihood of excess fat storage.

5. **Strategic Meal Timing:**

Distribute calories strategically throughout the day, with an emphasis on consuming a larger portion of calories around periods of increased activity. This aligns with the body's natural energy demands and helps optimize metabolism.

6. **Hydration is Key:**

Adequate hydration is crucial for metabolic processes and overall health. Drinking water before meals can also contribute to a sense of fullness, preventing overeating.

7. **Nutrient-Dense Foods:**

Choose nutrient-dense foods rich in vitamins, minerals, and antioxidants. Prioritize whole, unprocessed foods such as fruits, vegetables, lean proteins, and healthy fats to ensure optimal nutritional intake.

8. **Limit Processed and Sugary Foods:**

Minimize the consumption of processed foods, sugary snacks, and refined carbohydrates. These can contribute to excess calorie intake and may lead to fat storage, particularly in endomorphs.

9. **Personalized Approach:**

Recognize that individual responses to various foods can vary. Experiment with different dietary approaches, and consider consulting with a nutrition professional to create a personalized nutrition plan that aligns with specific preferences and requirements.

10. **Consistency and Patience:**

Consistency is key in endomorphic nutrition. Changes may take time, and it's essential to be patient while adopting a sustainable and balanced approach to achieve long-term health and fitness goals.

## The Role of Nutrient Timing in Boosting Metabolism

Nutrient timing plays a crucial role in boosting metabolism, and understanding when to consume specific nutrients can significantly impact energy utilization, muscle development, and overall metabolic efficiency. For individuals with an endomorphic body type, optimizing nutrient timing becomes particularly relevant in supporting their unique metabolic profile. Here's an exploration of the role of nutrient timing in boosting metabolism:

1. **Pre-Workout Nutrition:**

Consuming a balanced meal or snack containing carbohydrates and protein before a workout provides the body with readily available energy. This helps enhance workout performance and can contribute to an increased calorie burn during exercise.

2. **Post-Workout Nutrition:**

The post-workout period is a critical window for replenishing glycogen stores and initiating muscle repair and growth. Consuming a combination of carbohydrates and protein within this timeframe helps optimize recovery, supporting metabolic processes.

3. **Protein Distribution Throughout the Day:**

Distributing protein intake evenly across meals supports muscle protein synthesis and helps maintain lean muscle mass. This is essential for endomorphs, as increased muscle mass contributes to a higher resting metabolic rate.

4. **Carbohydrate Timing:**

Timing carbohydrate intake around periods of increased activity, such as during workouts or in the morning, can help regulate blood sugar levels. This strategic approach minimizes the likelihood of excess glucose being stored as fat.

5. **Meal Frequency:**

Consuming smaller, well-balanced meals throughout the day maintains a steady influx of nutrients. This approach can prevent energy slumps, optimize metabolism, and reduce the risk of overeating during larger meals.

6. **Evening Nutrition:**

While there is no strict rule against consuming nutrients in the evening, focusing on protein and fiber-rich foods can promote a feeling of fullness and stabilize blood sugar levels. This can be particularly beneficial for individuals with endomorphic traits prone to nighttime snacking.

### 7. **Hydration Timing:**

Staying adequately hydrated is vital for metabolism. Consuming water before meals can contribute to a sense of fullness, potentially reducing overall caloric intake.

### 8. **Balanced Nutrient Intake:**

Each meal should ideally include a balance of carbohydrates, proteins, and healthy fats. This combination provides sustained energy, promotes satiety, and supports various metabolic functions.

By strategically timing nutrient intake, individuals with an endomorphic body type can optimize their metabolism. This approach helps manage blood sugar levels, promotes efficient energy utilization, and supports the body's muscle-building and repair processes. Tailoring nutrient timing to individual needs and activity levels can contribute to a more effective and sustainable approach to metabolism enhancement.

## Meal Frequency and Portion Control Strategies

Meal frequency and portion control strategies are essential components of a nutritional approach, particularly for individuals with an endomorphic body type. These strategies can help regulate energy intake, manage blood sugar levels, and support overall metabolic health. Here are key considerations for meal frequency and portion control:

## 1. Meal Frequency Strategies:

**Frequent, Smaller Meals:**

Consuming smaller, balanced meals throughout the day, typically every 3-4 hours, helps maintain steady blood sugar levels and prevents excessive hunger. This approach can support a more consistent metabolic rate.

**Include Snacks:**

Incorporating nutritious snacks between main meals can curb hunger, prevent overeating during the next meal, and provide a constant source of energy throughout the day.

**Breakfast Importance:**

Starting the day with a well-balanced breakfast kickstarts metabolism and sets a positive tone for the rest of the day. Include a mix of protein, carbohydrates, and healthy fats for sustained energy.

**Pre-Workout and Post-Workout Nutrition:**

Timing meals or snacks around workouts is crucial. A pre-workout meal provides energy, while a post-workout meal supports recovery and muscle synthesis.

**Evening Meals:**

Distributing calories more evenly throughout the day and reducing the size of the evening meal may be beneficial for those with endomorphic traits, as it aligns with the body's natural circadian rhythms and may support better blood sugar control.

## 2. Portion Control Strategies:

**Use Smaller Plates:**

Opting for smaller plates can create the illusion of a fuller plate, promoting satisfaction with smaller portions.

**Mindful Eating:**

Paying attention to hunger and fullness cues helps prevent overeating. Eat slowly, savoring each bite, and pause between bites to gauge satiety.

**Pre-Portion Snacks:**

Pre-portioning snacks into smaller servings helps avoid mindless grazing and promotes portion control.

**Balance Macronutrients:**

Include a balance of protein, carbohydrates, and fats in each meal. This not only provides essential nutrients but also supports feelings of fullness.

**Hydrate Before Meals:**

Drinking water before meals can help create a feeling of fullness, preventing overconsumption of calories.

**Listen to Hunger Signals:**

Eat when hungry and stop when satisfied. Tuning into natural hunger and fullness cues promotes a healthier relationship with food.

**Plan and Prepare:**

Planning meals and preparing appropriate portion sizes can prevent the temptation to overeat or rely on less nutritious options.

Adopting these meal frequency and portion control strategies supports a balanced and sustainable approach to nutrition. For individuals with endomorphic traits, these practices can be particularly beneficial in managing weight, optimizing metabolism, and fostering overall well-being.

## Chapter 4

## Resetting Metabolic Workout Protocols

### Exercise Routines for Endomorphic Bodies

Creating a tailored exercise routine for individuals with endomorphic bodies involves a combination of cardiovascular exercises, strength training, and flexibility workouts. Below is a sample exercise routine with step-by-step instructions. Remember to warm up before starting any exercise and consult with a fitness professional or healthcare provider if you have any existing health conditions.

### Cardiovascular Exercise:

**1. Brisk Walking or Jogging:**

**Duration:** 30 minutes

**Steps:**

- Start with a 5-minute brisk walk to warm up.
- Gradually increase the pace to a moderate jog for 20 minutes.
- Finish with a 5-minute cooldown walk.

2. **High-Intensity Interval Training (HIIT):**

**Duration:** 20 minutes

**Steps:**

- Warm up for 5 minutes with light cardio.
- Alternate between 30 seconds of high-intensity exercises (e.g., jumping jacks, burpees) and 30 seconds of rest.

- Repeat the cycle for the entire duration.

**Strength Training:**

1. **Full-Body Strength Workout:**

**Frequency:** 2-3 times per week

**Steps:**

1. **Squats:**
   - Stand with feet shoulder-width apart.
   - Lower into a squat, keeping knees behind toes.
   - Perform 3 sets of 12 reps.

2. **Push-Ups:**
   - Start in a plank position.
   - Lower the chest towards the floor.

- Perform 3 sets of 10-12 reps.

3. **Dumbbell Rows:**

    - Hold a dumbbell in each hand, hinge at the hips, and row.
    - Perform 3 sets of 12 reps per arm.

## Flexibility and Mobility:

1. **Yoga Session:**

**Duration:** 20 minutes

**Steps:**

- Follow a beginner's yoga routine focusing on stretching and flexibility.
- Include poses like downward dog, cobra, and child's pose.

## Abdominal Training:

1. **Core Workout:**

**Frequency:** 2-3 times per week

**Steps:**

1. **Planks:**
   - Hold a plank position for 30-60 seconds.
   - Repeat for 3 sets.

2. **Russian Twists:**
   - Sit on the floor, lean back slightly, and twist your torso.
   - Perform 3 sets of 20 twists.

3. **Leg Raises:**
   - Lie on your back and lift your legs towards the ceiling.

- Perform 3 sets of 15-20 reps.

**Post-Workout Recovery:**

1. **Stretching Routine:**

**Duration:** 10 minutes

**Steps:**

- Focus on stretching major muscle groups.
- Include stretches for hamstrings, quadriceps, chest, and shoulders.

**Consistency and Progress:**

1. **Weekly Progression:**

**Steps:**

- Increase the intensity or duration of cardiovascular exercises gradually each week.

- Gradually increase the weight or resistance in strength training.

**Holistic Approach:**

1. **Mindful Practices:**

**Steps:**

- Incorporate mindfulness or stress-reducing activities such as deep breathing or meditation.

**Professional Guidance:**

1. **Consultation:**

**Steps:**

- Consider consulting with a fitness professional for personalized guidance and adjustments.

**Note:**

- Listen to your body and modify exercises as needed.
- Stay hydrated and maintain proper nutrition for optimal results.
- Adequate sleep is crucial for recovery and overall well-being.

Adjust the intensity and duration based on your fitness level and gradually progress over time. Consistency is key, and it's essential to enjoy the process of improving your overall fitness and well-being.

## High-Intensity Interval Training (HIIT) for Metabolic Acceleration

High-intensity interval Training (HIIT) is an effective workout method for metabolic acceleration, promoting calorie burn, and improving cardiovascular fitness. Here's a sample HIIT workout with step-by-step instructions. Always warm up before starting any high-intensity exercise, and consult with a fitness professional or healthcare provider if you have any existing health conditions.

**HIIT Workout for Metabolic Acceleration:**

**Warm-Up:**

- Perform a 5-10 minute dynamic warm-up, including exercises like jumping jacks, high knees, arm circles, and bodyweight squats.

**Workout:**

Perform each exercise at maximum effort for 30 seconds, followed by 30 seconds of rest. Complete the circuit for 3 rounds.

**1. Jumping Jacks:**

- Jump feet out while raising arms overhead.

- Land with feet together and arms at the sides.

**2. Burpees:**

- Start with a squat position, hands on the floor.
- Jump your feet back into a plank, and perform a push-up.
- Jump feet back towards hands, then explode into a jump.

**3. Mountain Climbers:**

- Start in a plank position.
- Drive knees towards the chest alternately.

**4. High Knees:**

- Run in place, lifting your knees as high as possible.

**5. Squat Jumps:**

- Perform a squat, then explode into a jump.

**6. Push-Ups:**

- Perform standard push-ups or modify as needed.

**7. Plank:**

- Hold a plank position, maintaining a straight line from head to heels.

**8. Jump Lunges:**

- Start in a lunge position, jump, and switch legs mid-air.

**9. Bicycle Crunches:**

- Lie on your back, and bring the opposite knee to the opposite elbow.

**10. Sprint in Place:**

- Run in place with maximum effort.

**Cool Down:**

- Perform a 5-10 minute cooldown consisting of light jogging or brisk walking, followed by static stretches for major muscle groups.

**Tips:**

- **Intensity:** Push yourself during the work intervals, aiming for maximum effort.

- **Form:** Maintain proper form to prevent injury.

- **Rest:** Rest for 30 seconds between exercises.

- **Modification:** Modify exercises based on fitness levels and any existing injuries.

**Frequency:**

Perform this HIIT workout 2-3 times per week, allowing at least one day of rest between sessions.

**Progression:**

As you build endurance, gradually increase work intervals or reduce rest periods.

**Note:**

Always listen to your body and adjust the intensity as needed. If you have any health concerns or conditions, consult with a healthcare professional before starting a new exercise program.

## Strength Training Techniques for Sculpting and Toning

Below is a strength training workout incorporating various techniques to help sculpt and tone different muscle groups.

Remember to warm up before starting and cool down after the workout. Adjust weights and repetitions based on your fitness level, and consult with a fitness professional or healthcare provider if you have any concerns.

**Warm-Up:**

Perform 5-10 minutes of light cardio (e.g., jogging in place, jumping jacks) followed by dynamic stretches for major muscle groups.

**Strength Training Workout:**

**1. Compound Exercises: Full Body Sculpting**

Perform each exercise for 3 sets of 10-12 repetitions.

1. Squats:

    - Stand with feet shoulder-width apart.
    - Lower into a squat, keeping knees behind toes.

- Return to the starting position.

2. Deadlifts:

    - Hold a barbell or dumbbell in front of you.

    - Hinge at the hips, lowering the weights toward the floor.

    - Keep the back straight and return to the starting position.

3. Bench Press:

    - Lie on a bench with a barbell or dumbbell.

    - Lower the weight to chest level and push back up.

4. Overhead Press:

    - Stand or sit with a barbell or dumbbell.

- Press the weight overhead, extending the arms fully.

## 2. High Repetition, Low Weight: Targeting Endurance

Perform each exercise for 3 sets of 15-20 repetitions.

1. Bicep Curls:
    - Hold dumbbells with palms facing forward.
    - Curl the weights toward your shoulders.
2. Tricep Dips:
    - Use parallel bars or a sturdy surface.
    - Lower and raise your body by bending and extending the elbows.

3. Lateral Raises:
    - Hold dumbbells at your sides.
    - Lift the weights to shoulder height.
4. Leg Extensions:
    - Use a leg extension machine or resistance bands.
    - Extend your legs against resistance.

**3. Supersetting: Sculpting with Efficiency**

Perform each superset without rest, then rest for 30 seconds between supersets.

1. Superset - Legs:
    - *Lunges:*
        - Step forward with one leg, lowering the back knee toward the floor.

- *Calf Raises:*
    - Rise onto the balls of your feet, lifting your heels.

2. Superset - Upper Body:
    - *Push-Ups:*
        - Perform standard or modified push-ups.
    - *Bent-Over Rows:*
        - Bend at the hips, and pull dumbbells toward your chest.

**4. Stability Ball Exercises: Core Focus**

Perform each exercise for 3 sets of 15-20 repetitions.

1. Stability Ball Plank:
    - Place your forearms on a stability ball, keeping your body in a straight line.
    - Hold the plank position.
2. Stability Ball Wall Squats:
    - Place the stability ball between your lower back and the wall.
    - Lower into a squat position.
3. Stability Ball Hamstring Curls:
    - Lie on your back with heels on the ball.
    - Lift your hips, pulling the ball toward you with your feet.

**Cool Down:**

Finish with 5-10 minutes of light cardio (e.g., brisk walking) and static stretches for major muscle groups.

**Tips:**

- The form is Critical: Maintain proper form throughout each exercise.

- Progress Gradually: Increase weights or resistance as you become stronger.

- Rest and Recovery: Allow at least 48 hours between strength training sessions for muscle recovery.

This workout targets various muscle groups for a comprehensive sculpting and toning effect. Adjust intensity and weights according to your fitness level and gradually progress over time.

## Chapter 5

## 4 weeks Meal Plan for Building Your Metabolic

## Week 1

Day 1:

- Breakfast: Scrambled eggs with spinach and whole-grain toast
- Snack: Greek yogurt with berries
- Lunch: Grilled chicken salad with mixed greens, tomatoes, and avocado
- Snack: Apple slices with almond butter
- Dinner: Baked salmon with quinoa and steamed broccoli

Day 2:

- Breakfast: Oatmeal with sliced bananas and a sprinkle of chia seeds

- Snack: Cottage cheese with pineapple chunks
- Lunch: Turkey and vegetable wrap with whole-grain tortilla
- Snack: Carrot sticks with hummus
- Dinner: Stir-fried tofu with brown rice and mixed vegetables

Day 3:

- Breakfast: Whole-grain toast with smashed avocado and poached eggs
- Snack: Handful of mixed nuts
- Lunch: Lentil soup with a side of whole-grain crackers
- Snack: Orange slices
- Dinner: Grilled shrimp with sweet potato wedges and asparagus

Day 4:

- Breakfast: Smoothie with spinach, banana, protein powder, and almond milk
- Snack: Cherry tomatoes with mozzarella cheese
- Lunch: Quinoa salad with chickpeas, cucumber, and feta cheese
- Snack: Pear slices with cottage cheese
- Dinner: Baked chicken breast with roasted Brussels sprouts and quinoa

Day 5:

- Breakfast: Greek yogurt parfait with granola and mixed berries
- Snack: Hard-boiled eggs

- Lunch: Whole-grain pasta with tomato sauce, lean ground turkey, and vegetables
- Snack: Mango slices
- Dinner: Beef stir-fry with brown rice and broccoli

Day 6:

- Breakfast: Whole-grain waffles with strawberries and a dollop of Greek yogurt
- Snack: Trail mix (almonds, walnuts, dried fruit)
- Lunch: Spinach and feta-stuffed chicken breast with quinoa
- Snack: Kiwi slices
- Dinner: Baked cod with sweet potato mash and green beans

Day 7:

- Breakfast: Veggie omelet with whole-grain toast
- Snack: Hummus with cucumber slices
- Lunch: Turkey and avocado lettuce wraps
- Snack: Pineapple chunks
- Dinner: Grilled steak with roasted root vegetables

**Week 2**

Day 8:

- Breakfast: Smoothie with spinach, banana, protein powder, and almond milk
- Snack: Handful of mixed nuts

- Lunch: Quinoa salad with grilled chicken, cherry tomatoes, and feta cheese

- Snack: Greek yogurt with a drizzle of honey

- Dinner: Baked salmon with lemon-dill sauce, sweet potato wedges, and steamed broccoli

Day 9:

- Breakfast: Whole-grain toast with smashed avocado, poached eggs, and a sprinkle of red pepper flakes

- Snack: Apple slices with almond butter

- Lunch: Lentil and vegetable stir-fry with brown rice

- Snack: Cottage cheese with pineapple chunks

- Dinner: Turkey chili with kidney beans, diced tomatoes, and a side of mixed greens

Day 10:

- Breakfast: Oatmeal with sliced strawberries, chia seeds, and a dollop of Greek yogurt
- Snack: Carrot and cucumber sticks with hummus
- Lunch: Spinach and feta-stuffed portobello mushrooms with a side of quinoa
- Snack: Orange slices
- Dinner: Grilled shrimp skewers with quinoa and roasted Brussels sprouts

Day 11:

- Breakfast: Whole-grain waffles with blueberries and a drizzle of maple syrup

- Snack: Trail mix (almonds, walnuts, dried cranberries)
- Lunch: Chicken Caesar salad with whole-grain croutons
- Snack: Mango slices
- Dinner: Baked cod with a side of asparagus and wild rice

Day 12:

- Breakfast: Scrambled tofu with sautéed spinach, tomatoes, and mushrooms
- Snack: Hard-boiled eggs
- Lunch: Whole-grain pasta primavera with mixed vegetables and grilled chicken
- Snack: Kiwi slices
- Dinner: Beef and vegetable kebabs with quinoa

Day 13:

- Breakfast: Greek yogurt parfait with granola and mixed berries
- Snack: Hummus with cucumber and bell pepper slices
- Lunch: Turkey and avocado wrap with whole-grain tortilla
- Snack: Pineapple and cottage cheese
- Dinner: Stir-fried tofu with broccoli, snap peas, and brown rice

Day 14:

- Breakfast: Veggie omelet with whole-grain toast
- Snack: Mixed berry smoothie with protein powder
- Lunch: Quinoa bowl with black beans, corn, cherry tomatoes, and guacamole

- Snack: Handful of almonds

- Dinner: Grilled steak with sweet potato mash and a side of green beans

## Week 3

Day 15:

- Breakfast: Acai bowl with granola, banana slices, and a sprinkle of chia seeds

- Snack: Handful of mixed berries

- Lunch: Shrimp and avocado salad with mixed greens, cherry tomatoes, and a light vinaigrette

- Snack: Greek yogurt with a handful of walnuts

- Dinner: Baked chicken breast with quinoa pilaf and roasted vegetables

Day 16:

- Breakfast: Whole-grain pancakes with raspberry compote and a dollop of coconut yogurt
- Snack: Sliced cucumber with tzatziki sauce
- Lunch: Lentil soup with a side of whole-grain crackers
- Snack: Orange slices
- Dinner: Grilled salmon with lemon-caper sauce, sweet potato wedges, and steamed broccoli

Day 17:

- Breakfast: Scrambled eggs with sautéed kale and cherry tomatoes
- Snack: Apple slices with almond butter

- Lunch: Quinoa-stuffed bell peppers with black beans, corn, and avocado
- Snack: Cottage cheese with pineapple chunks
- Dinner: Turkey and vegetable stir-fry with brown rice

Day 18:

- Breakfast: Chia seed pudding with mixed berries and a drizzle of honey
- Snack: Handful of mixed nuts
- Lunch: Chicken and vegetable curry with basmati rice
- Snack: Mango slices
- Dinner: Baked cod with a side of quinoa and roasted Brussels sprouts

Day 19:

- Breakfast: Whole-grain toast with smoked salmon, cream cheese, and capers
- Snack: Carrot and bell pepper sticks with hummus
- Lunch: Spinach and feta-stuffed chicken breast with quinoa
- Snack: Kiwi slices
- Dinner: Beef and vegetable kebabs with wild rice

Day 20:

- Breakfast: Greek yogurt parfait with granola, mixed berries, and a sprinkle of flaxseeds
- Snack: Trail mix (almonds, dried cranberries, pumpkin seeds)

- Lunch: Turkey and vegetable wrap with whole-grain tortilla
- Snack: Pineapple and cottage cheese
- Dinner: Stir-fried tofu with broccoli and brown rice

Day 21:

- Breakfast: Acai bowl with granola, banana slices, and a drizzle of honey
- Snack: Handful of mixed berries
- Lunch: Grilled shrimp and quinoa salad with mixed greens, cherry tomatoes, and avocado
- Snack: Greek yogurt with a handful of almonds
- Dinner: Baked chicken thighs with sweet potato wedges and steamed broccoli

## Week 4

Day 22:

- Breakfast: Whole-grain pancakes with blueberry compote and a dollop of coconut yogurt
- Snack: Sliced cucumber with tzatziki sauce
- Lunch: Lentil soup with a side of whole-grain crackers
- Snack: Orange slices
- Dinner: Grilled salmon with mango salsa, quinoa, and roasted Brussels sprouts

Day 23:

- Breakfast: Scrambled eggs with sautéed spinach and cherry tomatoes
- Snack: Apple slices with almond butter

- Lunch: Quinoa-stuffed bell peppers with black beans, corn, and avocado
- Snack: Cottage cheese with pineapple chunks
- Dinner: Turkey and vegetable stir-fry with brown rice

Day 24:

- Breakfast: Chia seed pudding with mixed berries and a drizzle of maple syrup
- Snack: Handful of mixed nuts
- Lunch: Chicken and vegetable curry with basmati rice
- Snack: Mango slices
- Dinner: Baked cod with a side of quinoa and roasted Brussels sprouts

Day 25:

- Breakfast: Whole-grain toast with smoked salmon, cream cheese, and capers
- Snack: Carrot and bell pepper sticks with hummus
- Lunch: Spinach and feta-stuffed chicken breast with quinoa
- Snack: Kiwi slices
- Dinner: Beef and vegetable kebabs with wild rice

Day 26:

- Breakfast: Greek yogurt parfait with granola, mixed berries, and a sprinkle of flaxseeds
- Snack: Trail mix (almonds, dried cranberries, pumpkin seeds)

- Lunch: Turkey and vegetable wrap with whole-grain tortilla

- Snack: Pineapple and cottage cheese

- Dinner: Stir-fried tofu with broccoli and brown rice

Day 27:

- Breakfast: Avocado toast with poached eggs and a sprinkle of red pepper flakes

- Snack: Handful of mixed berries

- Lunch: Quinoa salad with grilled chicken, cherry tomatoes, and feta cheese

- Snack: Greek yogurt with a drizzle of honey

- Dinner: Baked salmon with lemon-dill sauce, sweet potato wedges, and steamed broccoli

Day 28:

- Breakfast: Smoothie with spinach, banana, protein powder, and almond milk
- Snack: Handful of mixed nuts
- Lunch: Quinoa-stuffed bell peppers with black beans, corn, and avocado
- Snack: Cottage cheese with pineapple chunks
- Dinner: Turkey chili with kidney beans, diced tomatoes, and a side of mixed greens

## Chapter 7

## Metabolic Breakfast Boosters Recipes

### Protein-Packed Omelet

Ingredients:

- 3 eggs
- Spinach
- Cherry tomatoes, diced
- Feta cheese
- Olive oil

Instructions:

1. Whisk eggs in a bowl.
2. Sauté spinach and tomatoes in olive oil.
3. Pour whisked eggs over the veggies and cook until set.

4. Sprinkle feta cheese on top and fold the omelet.

Nutritional Benefits:

- High protein content supports muscle health.
- Spinach provides iron and vitamins.
- Tomatoes offer antioxidants.

**Quinoa Breakfast Bowl**

Ingredients:

- Cooked quinoa
- Greek yogurt
- Mixed berries (blueberries, strawberries)
- Almonds, chopped
- Honey

Instructions:

1. Mix cooked quinoa with Greek yogurt.
2. Top with mixed berries and chopped almonds.
3. Drizzle with honey.

Nutritional Benefits:

- Quinoa provides protein and fiber.
- Greek yogurt adds probiotics.
- Berries offer antioxidants.

## Avocado Toast with Poached Eggs

Ingredients:

- Whole-grain bread
- Avocado
- Eggs
- Red pepper flakes

- Salt and pepper

Instructions:

1. Toast whole-grain bread.
2. Mash avocado and spread on the toast.
3. Poach eggs and place on top.
4. Sprinkle with red pepper flakes, salt, and pepper.

Nutritional Benefits:

- Healthy fats from avocado.
- Eggs provide protein.
- Whole-grain bread offers fiber.

**Chia Seed Pudding Parfait**

Ingredients:

- Chia seeds
- Almond milk

- Greek yogurt
- Mixed berries
- Granola

Instructions:

1. Mix chia seeds with almond milk and let it sit overnight.
2. Layer chia pudding with Greek yogurt, berries, and granola.

Nutritional Benefits:

- Chia seeds provide omega-3 fatty acids.
- Greek yogurt offers protein.
- Berries contribute antioxidants.

## Spinach and Mushroom Breakfast Wrap

Ingredients:

- Whole-grain tortilla

- Eggs
- Spinach
- Mushrooms, sliced
- Cheese (optional)

Instructions:

1. Scramble eggs and cook with spinach and mushrooms.
2. Fill a whole-grain tortilla with the mixture.
3. Add cheese if desired and wrap it up.

Nutritional Benefits:

- Spinach and mushrooms provide vitamins.
- Whole-grain tortilla adds fiber.

## Blueberry Protein Smoothie

Ingredients:

- Blueberries
- Protein powder
- Almond milk
- Banana
- Chia seeds

Instructions:

1. Blend blueberries, protein powder, almond milk, banana, and chia seeds.

Nutritional Benefits:

- Blueberries offer antioxidants.
- Protein powder supports muscle health.
- Chia seeds provide omega-3s.

## Sweet Potato Hash with Turkey Sausage

Ingredients:

- Sweet potatoes, grated
- Turkey sausage, crumbled
- Red bell pepper, diced
- Onion, diced
- Olive oil

Instructions:

1. Sauté sweet potatoes, turkey sausage, bell pepper, and onion in olive oil.
2. Cook until sweet potatoes are tender.

Nutritional Benefits:

- Sweet potatoes provide complex carbs.
- Turkey sausage offers lean protein.
- Bell pepper adds vitamins.

## Cottage Cheese and Pineapple Bowl

Ingredients:

- Cottage cheese
- Pineapple chunks
- Walnuts, chopped
- Honey

Instructions:

1. Mix cottage cheese with pineapple chunks.
2. Top with chopped walnuts and a drizzle of honey.

Nutritional Benefits:

- Cottage cheese provides protein.
- Pineapple offers vitamins and enzymes.
- Walnuts add healthy fats.

## Egg and Veggie Breakfast Burrito

Ingredients:

- Whole-grain tortilla
- Eggs
- Bell peppers, diced
- Black beans
- Salsa

Instructions:

1. Scramble eggs and cook with diced bell peppers.
2. Fill a whole-grain tortilla with the egg mixture and black beans.
3. Top with salsa.

Nutritional Benefits:

- Bell peppers provide vitamins.
- Black beans offer fiber and protein.

- Whole-grain tortilla adds complex carbs.

## Peanut Butter Banana Toast

Ingredients:

- Whole-grain bread
- Peanut butter
- Banana, sliced
- Chia seeds

Instructions:

1. Toast whole-grain bread.
2. Spread peanut butter on the toast.
3. Top with banana slices and chia seeds.

Nutritional Benefits:

- Peanut butter provides protein.
- Banana offers potassium.
- Chia seeds add omega-3s.

## Salmon and Avocado Bagel

Ingredients:

- Whole-grain bagel
- Smoked salmon
- Avocado, sliced
- Cream cheese (optional)
- Dill

Instructions:

1. Toast a whole-grain bagel.
2. Spread cream cheese (if using).
3. Layer with smoked salmon, and avocado slices, and sprinkle with dill.

Nutritional Benefits:

- Salmon provides omega-3 fatty acids.
- Avocado adds healthy fats.

- Whole-grain bagel offers fiber.

## Mango Coconut Overnight Oats

Ingredients:

- Rolled oats
- Almond milk
- Mango, diced
- Coconut flakes
- Chopped nuts

Instructions:

1. Mix rolled oats with almond milk and let it sit overnight.
2. Top with diced mango, coconut flakes, and chopped nuts.

Nutritional Benefits:

- Oats offer fiber.

- Mango provides vitamins and antioxidants.
- Coconut adds healthy fats.

**Turkey and Spinach Breakfast Muffins**

Ingredients:

- Ground turkey
- Eggs
- Spinach, chopped
- Cherry tomatoes, diced
- Feta cheese

Instructions:

1. Cook ground turkey and mix with chopped spinach and diced tomatoes.
2. Whisk eggs and pour over the turkey mixture.

3. Add feta cheese and bake in muffin cups.

Nutritional Benefits:

- Turkey provides lean protein.
- Spinach offers vitamins.
- Feta cheese adds flavor and calcium.

**Raspberry Almond Chia Pudding**

Ingredients:

- Chia seeds
- Almond milk
- Raspberries
- Almonds, sliced
- Maple syrup

Instructions:

1. Mix chia seeds with almond milk and let it sit overnight.
2. Layer chia pudding with raspberries, sliced almonds, and a drizzle of maple syrup.

Nutritional Benefits:

- Chia seeds provide omega-3s.
- Raspberries offer antioxidants.
- Almonds add healthy fats.

**Green Tea Smoothie**

Ingredients:

- Green tea (brewed and cooled)
- Greek yogurt
- Pineapple chunks
- Spinach

- Honey

Instructions:

1. Blend brewed and cooled green tea with Greek yogurt, pineapple chunks, spinach, and honey.

Nutritional Benefits:

- Green tea provides antioxidants.
- Greek yogurt adds protein.
- Spinach offers vitamins.

## Chapter 8

## Metabolic Lunchtime Power Recipes

### Grilled Chicken and Quinoa Salad

Ingredients:

- Grilled chicken breast
- Quinoa
- Mixed greens
- Cherry tomatoes, halved
- Cucumber, sliced
- Balsamic vinaigrette

Instructions:

1. Cook quinoa according to package instructions.
2. Grill chicken and slice.

3. Assemble a salad with mixed greens, quinoa, grilled chicken, tomatoes, and cucumber.

4. Drizzle with balsamic vinaigrette.

Nutritional Benefits:

- Chicken provides lean protein.
- Quinoa offers complex carbs.
- Veggies add vitamins and fiber.

**Salmon and Avocado Wrap**

Ingredients:

- Grilled salmon
- Whole-grain wrap
- Avocado, sliced
- Spinach
- Greek yogurt sauce

Instructions:

1. Grill salmon and flake it.
2. Lay out a whole-grain wrap and add salmon, sliced avocado, spinach, and Greek yogurt sauce.
3. Roll it up and enjoy.

Nutritional Benefits:

- Salmon provides omega-3s.
- Avocado adds healthy fats.
- Whole-grain wrap offers fiber.

## Mediterranean Chickpea Salad

Ingredients:

- Chickpeas, canned and rinsed
- Cherry tomatoes, halved
- Cucumber, diced

- Red onion, finely chopped
- Feta cheese
- Olive oil and lemon dressing

Instructions:

1. Combine chickpeas, tomatoes, cucumber, red onion, and feta cheese.
2. Toss with olive oil and lemon dressing.

Nutritional Benefits:

- Chickpeas provide protein and fiber.
- Veggies offer vitamins.
- Feta cheese adds calcium.

**Turkey and Quinoa Stuffed Peppers**

Ingredients:

- Ground turkey
- Quinoa

- Bell peppers
- Black beans, canned and rinsed
- Salsa

Instructions:

1. Cook quinoa and brown ground turkey.
2. Mix with black beans and salsa.
3. Stuff bell peppers with the mixture and bake.

Nutritional Benefits:

- Turkey offers lean protein.
- Quinoa provides complex carbs.
- Peppers add vitamins.

## Whole-grain pasta with Pesto and Veggies

Ingredients:

- Whole-grain pasta

- Pesto sauce
- Cherry tomatoes, halved
- Broccoli, chopped
- Parmesan cheese

Instructions:

1. Cook whole-grain pasta.
2. Mix with pesto sauce, cherry tomatoes, and broccoli.
3. Top with Parmesan cheese.

Nutritional Benefits:

- Whole-grain pasta offers fiber.
- Veggies provide vitamins.
- Pesto adds flavor.

## Shrimp and Quinoa Bowl

Ingredients:

- Shrimp, peeled and deveined
- Quinoa
- Avocado, sliced
- Black beans, canned and rinsed
- Lime vinaigrette

Instructions:

1. Cook quinoa and sauté shrimp.
2. Assemble a bowl with quinoa, shrimp, sliced avocado, and black beans.
3. Drizzle with lime vinaigrette.

Nutritional Benefits:

- Shrimp provides protein.
- Quinoa offers complex carbs.

- Avocado adds healthy fats.

## Vegetarian Chickpea Stir-Fry

Ingredients:

- Chickpeas, canned and rinsed
- Broccoli, florets
- Carrots, sliced
- Snap peas
- Soy sauce

Instructions:

1. Sauté chickpeas, broccoli, carrots, and snap peas.
2. Add soy sauce and stir until veggies are tender.

Nutritional Benefits:

- Chickpeas offer protein and fiber.

- Veggies provide vitamins.
- Soy sauce adds flavor.

**Tuna Salad Stuffed Avocado**

Ingredients:

- Canned tuna, drained
- Avocado, halved
- Cherry tomatoes, diced
- Red onion, finely chopped
- Greek yogurt

Instructions:

1. Mix tuna with cherry tomatoes, red onion, and Greek yogurt.
2. Scoop the mixture into halved avocados.

Nutritional Benefits:

- Tuna provides protein.
- Avocado adds healthy fats.
- Greek yogurt offers probiotics.

**Eggplant and Lentil Curry**

Ingredients:

- Eggplant, diced
- Lentils, cooked
- Tomatoes, diced
- Coconut milk
- Curry spices

Instructions:

1. Sauté eggplant and add cooked lentils and tomatoes.

2. Pour in coconut milk and add curry spices.

3. Simmer until eggplant is tender.

Nutritional Benefits:

- Lentils offer protein and fiber.
- Eggplant provides vitamins.
- Coconut milk adds flavor and healthy fats.

## Chicken and Vegetable Quinoa Bowl

Ingredients:

- Grilled chicken breast, sliced
- Quinoa
- Zucchini, sliced
- Bell peppers, diced
- Teriyaki sauce

Instructions:

1. Cook quinoa and grill chicken.
2. Sauté zucchini and bell peppers with teriyaki sauce.
3. Assemble a bowl with quinoa, grilled chicken, and veggies.

Nutritional Benefits:

- Chicken provides protein.
- Quinoa offers complex carbs.
- Veggies add vitamins.

**Sweet Potato and Black Bean Quesadilla**

Ingredients:

- Sweet potato, grated
- Black beans, canned and rinsed
- Whole-grain tortillas

- Cheese
- Salsa

Instructions:

1. Mix grated sweet potato with black beans.
2. Fill a whole-grain tortilla with the mixture and cheese.
3. Cook until cheese melts, then serve with salsa.

Nutritional Benefits:

- Sweet potato provides complex carbs.
- Black beans offer protein and fiber.
- Whole-grain tortilla adds fiber.

## Caprese Salad with Grilled Chicken

Ingredients:

- Grilled chicken breast, sliced

- Tomatoes, sliced
- Fresh mozzarella, sliced
- Basil leaves
- Balsamic glaze

Instructions:

1. Arrange sliced tomatoes, mozzarella, and grilled chicken on a plate.
2. Top with fresh basil leaves and drizzle with balsamic glaze.

Nutritional Benefits:

- Chicken provides protein.
- Tomatoes offer vitamins.
- Mozzarella adds calcium.

## Lentil and Vegetable Soup

Ingredients:

- Lentils, cooked
- Carrots, diced
- Celery, sliced
- Spinach, chopped
- Vegetable broth

Instructions:

1. Sauté carrots and celery, then add cooked lentils and vegetable broth.
2. Simmer until veggies are tender, then stir in chopped spinach.

Nutritional Benefits:

- Lentils offer protein and fiber.
- Veggies provide vitamins.
- Vegetable broth adds flavor.

## Turkey and Quinoa Stuffed Acorn Squash

Ingredients:

- Ground turkey
- Quinoa
- Acorn squash, halved
- Cranberries
- Pecans, chopped

Instructions:

1. Cook quinoa and brown ground turkey.
2. Mix with cranberries and pecans.
3. Stuff acorn squash halves and bake.

Nutritional Benefits:

- Turkey provides lean protein.
- Quinoa offers complex carbs.
- Acorn squash adds vitamins.

## Asian-Inspired Tofu Stir-Fry

Ingredients:

- Tofu cubed
- Broccoli, florets
- Snow peas
- Bell peppers, sliced
- Soy sauce

Instructions:

1. Sauté tofu, broccoli, snow peas, and bell peppers.
2. Add soy sauce and stir until veggies are tender.

Nutritional Benefits:

- Tofu offers plant-based protein.
- Veggies provide vitamins.
- Soy sauce adds flavor.

## Chapter 9

## Metabolic Dinner Delights Recipes

### Grilled Salmon with Lemon-Dill Sauce

Ingredients:

- Salmon fillets
- Lemon juice
- Fresh dill, chopped
- Olive oil
- Garlic, minced

Instructions:

1. Season salmon with lemon juice, fresh dill, olive oil, and minced garlic.
2. Grill until salmon is cooked through.

Nutritional Benefits:

- Salmon provides omega-3 fatty acids.

- Lemon adds vitamin C.

- Dill offers antioxidants.

## Quinoa and Vegetable Stuffed Bell Peppers

Ingredients:

- Quinoa

- Bell peppers, halved

- Black beans, canned and rinsed

- Corn kernels

- Salsa

Instructions:

1. Cook quinoa and mix with black beans, corn, and salsa.

2. Stuff bell pepper halves with the mixture and bake until the peppers are tender.

Nutritional Benefits:

- Quinoa offers protein and complex carbs.
- Bell peppers provide vitamins.
- Black beans add fiber.

**Chicken and Broccoli Stir-Fry**

Ingredients:

- Chicken breast, sliced
- Broccoli florets
- Soy sauce
- Ginger, minced
- Brown rice

Instructions:

1. Sauté chicken and broccoli in soy sauce and minced ginger.

2. Serve over cooked brown rice.

Nutritional Benefits:

- Chicken provides protein.
- Broccoli offers vitamins.
- Brown rice adds fiber.

**Vegetarian Lentil Soup**

Ingredients:

- Lentils, cooked
- Carrots, diced
- Celery, sliced
- Onion, chopped
- Vegetable broth

Instructions:

1. Sauté carrots, celery, and onion, then add cooked lentils and vegetable broth.

2. Simmer until veggies are tender.

Nutritional Benefits:

- Lentils offer protein and fiber.
- Veggies provide vitamins.
- Vegetable broth adds flavor.

## Mushroom and Spinach Stuffed Chicken Breast

Ingredients:

- Chicken breast
- Mushrooms, sliced
- Spinach, chopped
- Garlic, minced

- Mozzarella cheese

Instructions:

1. Butterfly chicken breast and stuff with sautéed mushrooms, spinach, garlic, and mozzarella.

2. Bake until chicken is cooked through.

Nutritional Benefits:

- Chicken provides protein.
- Spinach offers vitamins.
- Mozzarella adds calcium.

## Sweet Potato and Chickpea Curry

Ingredients:

- Sweet potatoes, diced
- Chickpeas, canned and rinsed
- Coconut milk

- Curry spices
- Basmati rice

Instructions:

1. Sauté sweet potatoes and chickpeas in coconut milk with curry spices.
2. Serve over cooked basmati rice.

Nutritional Benefits:

- Sweet potatoes offer complex carbs.
- Chickpeas provide protein and fiber.
- Coconut milk adds flavor.

**Baked Cod with Mediterranean Salsa**

Ingredients:

- Cod fillets
- Tomatoes, diced
- Kalamata olives, sliced

- Red onion, finely chopped
- Olive oil

Instructions:

1. Season cod with olive oil and bake until cooked through.
2. Top with a salsa made from diced tomatoes, olives, and red onion.

Nutritional Benefits:

- Cod provides lean protein.
- Tomatoes offer vitamins.
- Olives add healthy fats.

**Vegetable and Tofu Stir-Fry**

Ingredients:

- Tofu cubed
- Broccoli florets

- Carrots, sliced
- Snap peas
- Soy sauce

Instructions:

1. Sauté tofu, broccoli, carrots, and snap peas.
2. Add soy sauce and stir until veggies are tender.

Nutritional Benefits:

- Tofu offers plant-based protein.
- Veggies provide vitamins.
- Soy sauce adds flavor.

**Spinach and Feta-Stuffed Chicken Thighs**

Ingredients:

- Chicken thighs

- Spinach, chopped
- Feta cheese
- Lemon juice
- Garlic, minced

Instructions:

1. Season chicken thighs with lemon juice and minced garlic.
2. Stuff with a mixture of chopped spinach and feta.
3. Bake until chicken is cooked through.

Nutritional Benefits:

- Chicken provides protein.
- Spinach offers vitamins.
- Feta adds flavor and calcium.

## Lemon Herb Grilled Shrimp

Ingredients:

- Shrimp, peeled and deveined
- Lemon zest
- Fresh herbs (such as parsley and thyme)
- Olive oil
- Garlic, minced

Instructions:

1. Marinate shrimp with lemon zest, fresh herbs, olive oil, and minced garlic.
2. Grill until shrimp are cooked.

Nutritional Benefits:

- Shrimp provides protein.
- Lemon adds vitamin C.
- Fresh herbs offer antioxidants.

## Veggie-Packed Turkey Chili

Ingredients:

- Ground turkey
- Kidney beans, canned and rinsed
- Tomatoes, diced
- Bell peppers, diced
- Chili spices

Instructions:

1. Brown ground turkey and add kidney beans, tomatoes, bell peppers, and chili spices.
2. Simmer until flavors meld.

Nutritional Benefits:

- Turkey provides protein.
- Kidney beans offer fiber.
- Veggies add vitamins.

## Cauliflower and Chickpea Curry

Ingredients:

- Cauliflower, florets
- Chickpeas, canned and rinsed
- Coconut milk
- Curry spices
- Basmati rice

Instructions:

1. Sauté cauliflower and chickpeas in coconut milk with curry spices.
2. Serve over cooked basmati rice.

Nutritional Benefits:

- Cauliflower provides vitamins.
- Chickpeas offer protein and fiber.
- Coconut milk adds flavor.

## Sesame Ginger Beef Stir-Fry

Ingredients:

- Beef strips
- Broccoli florets
- Snap peas
- Bell peppers, sliced
- Sesame ginger sauce

Instructions:

1. Sauté beef strips, broccoli, snap peas, and bell peppers.
2. Add sesame ginger sauce and stir until beef is cooked and veggies are tender.

Nutritional Benefits:

- Beef provides protein.
- Veggies offer vitamins.
- Sesame ginger sauce adds flavor.

## Pesto Zoodles with Grilled Chicken

Ingredients:

- Zucchini spiralized
- Grilled chicken breast, sliced
- Cherry tomatoes, halved
- Pesto sauce
- Parmesan cheese

Instructions:

1. Sauté zucchini noodles until tender.
2. Toss with grilled chicken, cherry tomatoes, pesto sauce, and Parmesan cheese.

Nutritional Benefits:

- Chicken provides protein.
- Zucchini offers vitamins.
- Pesto adds flavor.

# Chapter 10

# Metabolic Snack Smart Recipes

## Almond Butter Banana Bites

Ingredients:

- Banana, sliced
- Almond butter
- Chia seeds

Instructions:

1. Spread almond butter on banana slices.
2. Sprinkle with chia seeds.

Nutritional Benefits:

- Banana provides potassium.
- Almond butter offers healthy fats.
- Chia seeds add omega-3s.

## Cucumber and Hummus

Ingredients:

- Cucumber, sliced
- Hummus

Instructions:

1. Dip cucumber slices into hummus.

Nutritional Benefits:

- Cucumber adds hydration.
- Hummus provides protein and healthy fats.

## Hard-Boiled Eggs with Avocado

Ingredients:

- Hard-boiled eggs
- Avocado, sliced
- Everything bagel seasoning

Instructions:

1. Slice hard-boiled eggs and top with avocado slices.
2. Sprinkle with everything bagel seasoning.

Nutritional Benefits:

- Eggs offer protein.
- Avocado adds healthy fats.
- Everything bagel seasoning adds flavor.

**Trail Mix**

Ingredients:

- Almonds
- Walnuts
- Dried cranberries
- Dark chocolate chips

Instructions:

1. Mix almonds, walnuts, dried cranberries, and dark chocolate chips.

Nutritional Benefits:

- Nuts provide healthy fats and protein.
- Dried cranberries offer antioxidants.
- Dark chocolate chips add a touch of sweetness.

**Apple Slices with Peanut Butter**

Ingredients:

- Apple, sliced
- Peanut butter

Instructions:

1. Dip apple slices into peanut butter.

Nutritional Benefits:

- Apple provides fiber.
- Peanut butter offers protein and healthy fats.

## Rice Cake with Cottage Cheese and Pineapple

Ingredients:

- Rice cake
- Cottage cheese
- Pineapple chunks

Instructions:

1. Spread cottage cheese on a rice cake.
2. Top with pineapple chunks.

Nutritional Benefits:

- Rice cake offers complex carbs.
- Cottage cheese provides protein.
- Pineapple adds vitamins.

## Kale Chips

Ingredients:

- Kale leaves, torn into pieces
- Olive oil
- Sea salt

Instructions:

1. Toss kale pieces with olive oil and sea salt.
2. Bake until crispy.

Nutritional Benefits:

- Kale offers vitamins and minerals.
- Olive oil adds healthy fats.

## Cherry Tomatoes with Mozzarella

Ingredients:

- Cherry tomatoes, halved

- Fresh mozzarella balls
- Basil leaves
- Balsamic glaze

Instructions:

1. Skewer cherry tomatoes, mozzarella balls, and basil leaves.
2. Drizzle with balsamic glaze.

Nutritional Benefits:

- Tomatoes offer vitamins.
- Mozzarella adds calcium.
- Basil provides antioxidants.

**Carrot Sticks with Hummus**

Ingredients:

- Carrot sticks
- Hummus

Instructions:

1. Dip carrot sticks into hummus.

Nutritional Benefits:

- Carrots provide beta-carotene.
- Hummus offers protein and healthy fats.

**Cottage Cheese and Mango Salsa**

Ingredients:

- Cottage cheese
- Mango, diced
- Red onion, finely chopped
- Cilantro, chopped

Instructions:

1. Mix cottage cheese with mango, red onion, and cilantro.

Nutritional Benefits:

- Cottage cheese provides protein.
- Mango offers vitamins and antioxidants.
- Cilantro adds flavor.

**Stuffed Dates with Almond Butter**

Ingredients:

- Medjool dates, pitted
- Almond butter
- Pecans, chopped

Instructions:

1. Fill dates with almond butter.
2. Sprinkle with chopped pecans.

Nutritional Benefits:

- Dates offer natural sweetness.

- Almond butter provides healthy fats and protein.

- Pecans add crunch and healthy fats.

**Whole Grain Crackers with Tuna Salad**

Ingredients:

- Whole grain crackers
- Canned tuna, drained
- Greek yogurt
- Dill, chopped

Instructions:

1. Mix tuna with Greek yogurt and chopped dill.
2. Spread on whole-grain crackers.

Nutritional Benefits:

- Whole grain crackers offer complex carbs.

- Tuna provides protein.
- Greek yogurt adds probiotics.

**Yogurt-Dipped Strawberries**

Ingredients:

- Strawberries, washed
- Greek yogurt
- Honey

Instructions:

1. Dip strawberries into Greek yogurt.
2. Drizzle with honey.

Nutritional Benefits:

- Strawberries offer vitamins and antioxidants.
- Greek yogurt provides protein.
- Honey adds sweetness.

**Pumpkin Seeds and Dried Apricots**

Ingredients:

- Pumpkin seeds
- Dried apricots, chopped

Instructions:

1. Mix pumpkin seeds with chopped dried apricots.

Nutritional Benefits:

- Pumpkin seeds offer protein and healthy fats.
- Dried apricots provide natural sweetness and vitamins.

## Chapter 11

## Conclusion

In conclusion, the Metabolic Diet plan and exercise for endomorphs represent a comprehensive and nuanced approach to addressing the unique metabolic characteristics of individuals with an endomorphic body type. This well-crafted program goes beyond the conventional one-size-fits-all dieting strategies, recognizing the diversity inherent in individual metabolisms and lifestyles.

One of the core strengths of the Metabolic Diet lies in its emphasis on personalization and flexibility. By acknowledging the inherent uniqueness of each endomorphic individual, the plan allows for adaptable dietary choices, macronutrient adjustments, and personalized meal timing. This individualized approach recognizes that no two bodies are identical, and as such, the program becomes a dynamic framework capable of accommodating a range of preferences and responses.

A pivotal aspect of this diet plan is its focus on achieving a balanced intake of macronutrients. By ensuring an equilibrium between proteins, carbohydrates, and fats, the plan not only supports the primary goal of fat loss but also promotes sustained energy levels and the preservation of lean muscle mass. This balance plays a crucial role in overall metabolic health, fostering an environment conducive to achieving and maintaining optimal body composition.

Strategic meal timing is another distinguishing feature of the Reset Diet. By aligning nutrient intake with the body's natural circadian rhythms, the plan maximizes the body's metabolic efficiency. This temporal synchronization enhances nutrient utilization, regulates insulin sensitivity, and optimizes energy expenditure, contributing to the overall effectiveness of the diet plan.

Beyond the realm of dietary recommendations, the Metabolic Diet integrates physical activity as an essential component of the program. Recognizing the symbiotic relationship between nutrition and exercise, the plan provides tailored workout suggestions, incorporating strength training, high-intensity interval training (HIIT), and targeted exercises designed specifically for endomorphic bodies. This holistic approach underscores the interconnectedness of nutrition and fitness in achieving optimal metabolic health.

Education is a cornerstone of the Reset Diet, empowering individuals with a deeper understanding of their metabolism, hormonal influences, and the impact of dietary choices. This knowledge equips participants with the tools to make informed decisions about their health beyond the structured plan, fostering a sense of autonomy and self-efficacy.

Moreover, the program encourages a mindset shift by celebrating not only numerical achievements on the scale but also non-scale victories. Recognizing improvements in energy levels, mood, sleep quality, and overall well-being reinforces the intrinsic value of the health journey, promoting a positive and sustainable approach to lifestyle changes.

In essence, the Reset Diet plan and exercise for endomorphs stand as a testament to the transformative potential of a personalized and knowledge-driven approach to nutrition and lifestyle. By embracing principles of balance, flexibility, and sustainability, this program provides individuals with a roadmap to reset their metabolism, achieve their fitness goals, and embark on a journey toward enduring health and vitality.

Made in United States
North Haven, CT
29 March 2024

50638875R00078